R.C. MORALES

Preventing Infections in PAP Equipment

Best practices for cleaning, disinfecting, and preventing cross-contamination, especially for users with weakened immune systems

Contents

Introduction

The world of medicine, though rich in complexity and innovation, has its share of paradoxes. Few tools in modern healthcare illustrate this better than Positive Airway Pressure (PAP) therapy. Designed to treat conditions like obstructive sleep apnea (OSA) and other respiratory disorders, PAP therapy holds the promise of transformative healing, yet its effectiveness depends not only on how the equipment works but on how well it's cared for. This book is dedicated to exploring that crucial aspect—how to protect the equipment, maintain its function, and, in doing so, safeguard the very health of those who rely on it.

What is PAP Therapy?

PAP therapy is a medical treatment designed to assist individuals with sleep-disordered breathing. At its core, PAP therapy delivers a continuous flow of air through a mask to keep the airway open during sleep, preventing the collapse that leads to interruptions in breathing. The "positive pressure" in the acronym refers to this continuous airflow, which ensures that a person's airway remains patent, preventing the dangerous pauses in breathing that characterize conditions like obstructive sleep apnea (OSA). Depending on the severity of the condition, there are different types of PAP devices, ranging from CPAP (Continuous Positive Airway Pressure) for simpler cases to Bi-

PAP (Bilevel Positive Airway Pressure) or APAP (Auto-titrating Positive Airway Pressure) for more complex needs.

This therapy is simple in concept but profound in its impact. It is the difference between a night of restless, disordered breathing and a night of restful, life-giving sleep. The devices themselves, while relatively small and unobtrusive, provide an essential function that enhances oxygenation, reduces daytime fatigue, and protects long-term cardiovascular health. For people with compromised immune systems or other chronic health conditions, PAP therapy can be a lifeline, dramatically improving their quality of life.

The Benefits of PAP Therapy

The benefits of PAP therapy extend far beyond simply improving sleep. For individuals with conditions like OSA, untreated, the consequences can be severe—ranging from chronic fatigue and increased risk of hypertension, stroke, or heart disease. Effective treatment with PAP not only alleviates these risks but can have a far-reaching impact on one's overall health.

Regular use of PAP therapy helps restore the natural rhythm of sleep, which in turn fosters a multitude of healing processes. From cognitive function to emotional well-being, the improvements are remarkable. Imagine waking up after a full, uninterrupted night of sleep—not just feeling more rested, but more energized, focused, and capable of managing life's demands. This is the power of PAP therapy, and it is a benefit not just to the body, but to the mind and spirit.

For individuals with weakened immune systems—those undergoing cancer treatments, living with autoimmune diseases, or managing chronic respiratory illnesses—the stakes are even higher. The restorative powers of sleep, combined with the consistent support of PAP therapy, offer these individuals a fighting chance against the further depletion of energy reserves and the onset of complications that could arise from sleep-disordered breathing. In fact, proper use of PAP therapy can strengthen the body's ability to fight infections and accelerate recovery, making it one of the most effective non-invasive treatments for those facing chronic health challenges.

PAP Therapy: Not Easy, But Rewarding

Despite its immense benefits, PAP therapy is not without its challenges. It's not simply a matter of setting up a machine and falling asleep. For many, there's a period of adjustment—getting used to wearing a mask over the face, adapting to the sensation of the constant airflow, and overcoming the initial discomfort of a new routine. But as with any worthwhile endeavor, persistence and care yield remarkable results.

The path to reaping the full benefits of PAP therapy requires commitment. Some individuals may struggle to make it through the first few nights. The mask might feel restrictive or awkward, or the sound of the machine may seem intrusive. For others, using the equipment requires significant adjustments in lifestyle. Traveling, for example, or managing the equipment in a busy household can pose logistical challenges. The therapy itself demands attention to detail—cleaning and maintenance, ensuring there are no obstructions in the tubing, and managing the mask to avoid irritation or infection.

For those with weakened immune systems, this maintenance becomes even more critical. Contamination of the equipment could lead to dangerous infections or exacerbate existing conditions. The process of cleaning, disinfecting, and managing cross-contamination becomes more than a simple hygiene task; it becomes an integral part of the therapy itself, an act of safeguarding the fragile balance of health that the PAP machine helps maintain.

But in the end, the rewards far outweigh the challenges. Those who stick with it find their health improving in ways they hadn't imagined. In time, PAP therapy becomes more than just a nightly routine; it becomes a foundation for better sleep, better health, and a better life.

The pages that follow will guide you through the essentials of proper care for PAP equipment, addressing common pitfalls and offering practical solutions to prevent cross-contamination and infections. We will explore best practices for cleaning and disinfecting your devices, with particular attention to the needs of those with compromised immune systems. With a little effort, diligence, and the right knowledge, the therapeutic benefits of PAP can be maximized, ensuring not just comfort but safety as well.

In the end, while the road may not always be easy, the rewards of PAP therapy are worth every step. The result is a life with better rest, better health, and better protection—one breath at a time.

1

Protecting Your Health with Careful Maintenance

E very night, your Positive Airway Pressure (PAP) equipment provides you with something precious— steady, reliable breath. For people living with conditions like sleep apnea or other breathing issues, this equipment can mean the difference between waking up refreshed and facing serious health challenges. But while these machines are powerful tools for healing, they can also carry risks if they're not properly maintained.

PAP equipment is a lifeline, but it's also a warm, moist environment—an ideal home for bacteria, mold, and viruses. For anyone, this can lead to unwanted health problems. For those with weaker immune systems, such as people undergoing cancer treatment, living with chronic illnesses, or managing autoimmune conditions, these risks are even more serious. Thankfully, preventing these problems isn't complicated. It's about building a simple routine that keeps your equipment clean, safe, and ready to support you.

Some people hesitate when it comes to cleaning their PAP machines. Maybe the manufacturer's instructions felt vague or overwhelming, or maybe life just gets busy. But neglecting this task can lead to infections, allergic reactions, or worse. This book is here to guide you, offering clear, practical steps to help you care for your equipment with confidence.

Each part of your PAP machine—whether it's the mask, tubing, or humidifier—needs attention. Cleaning removes dirt, oil, and particles that build up with regular use. Disinfecting goes a step further, targeting germs that you can't see. Together, these steps help make sure your PAP equipment is working for you, not against you.

If your immune system is weakened, taking these steps is even more critical. Regular cleaning and disinfecting are essential, but so is understanding how to protect yourself from cross-contamination if you share living spaces or have caregivers who assist with your equipment. It might sound like a lot at first, but it quickly becomes second nature—just a small part of your routine that makes a big difference.

This book isn't just about the mechanics of cleaning; it's about empowering you. Proper maintenance doesn't take much time, but the benefits are huge: peace of mind, better health, and equipment that supports you fully. With every step, you're taking control, ensuring that your PAP machine stays a source of healing, not harm.

You deserve to feel safe and supported in your therapy. Let this guide walk with you, helping you create a maintenance routine that's simple, effective, and tailored to your needs. Together, we'll turn this lifeline into a source of ongoing comfort and health.

2

Understanding the Importance of Proper PAP Equipment Maintenance

Positive Airway Pressure (PAP) therapy has transformed lives, offering relief to those struggling with sleep apnea, chronic breathing problems, and other respiratory conditions. By delivering a steady stream of air, PAP devices keep airways open, ensuring restful sleep and improved health. The most common equipment includes a mask that fits over the nose or mouth, a machine that generates airflow, tubing to connect the two, and sometimes a humidifier to make the air more comfortable to breathe. These parts work together seamlessly—until they don't.

Like any tool you rely on daily, your PAP equipment needs care. Each time you use it, oils from your skin, moisture from your breath, and airborne particles collect on its surfaces. Left unattended, these deposits create an environment where bacteria, mold, and viruses can thrive. For people with strong immune systems, this can cause minor irritations or infections.

But for those with weakened immunity, the consequences can be far more serious, including severe respiratory infections or allergic reactions.

The risks don't stop there. Dirty equipment can also impact the effectiveness of your therapy. A clogged filter or obstructed tubing can reduce airflow, while a buildup of germs inside the device can lead to unpleasant odors and even damage over time. What should be a source of comfort and healing becomes a potential source of harm.

The good news is that these problems are entirely preventable. Effective maintenance of your PAP equipment has three main goals: to protect your health, to ensure your therapy works as it should, and to extend the life of your device. Regular cleaning and disinfecting remove harmful germs and debris, keeping the air you breathe clean and safe. Proper care also helps your equipment perform at its best, delivering the consistent airflow your body depends on each night.

Maintaining your PAP equipment isn't just about following instructions—it's about understanding why these steps matter and making them a habit. With just a bit of daily attention, you can keep your equipment clean, safe, and effective. It's an investment in your therapy, your health, and your peace of mind.

3

Step-by-Step Guide to Cleaning and Disinfecting PAP Equipment

Caring for your PAP equipment doesn't have to be complicated. With a simple routine and the right techniques, you can ensure your device stays clean, safe, and effective. This guide walks you through daily cleaning, weekly maintenance, and specialized sterilization methods for high-risk situations.

Daily Cleaning Practices for PAP Equipment

Start every day by giving your PAP equipment a quick, thorough clean. Begin by disconnecting the mask, tubing, and humidifier chamber from the machine. Wash the mask and tubing in warm water with mild, unscented soap. Gently scrub to remove oils, moisture, and particles that accumulate during use. Rinse thoroughly to ensure no soap residue remains, as it can irritate your skin or respiratory system. If your machine has a humidifier, empty any leftover water, rinse the chamber, and let it air-dry to prevent bacteria or mold from forming.

Dry all components completely before reassembling them. Moisture left inside tubing or the mask can create a breeding ground for germs. Using a soft, clean cloth can speed up drying, but always let the equipment air out fully in a clean area away from direct sunlight.

Weekly Cleaning and Disinfection Procedures

Weekly care goes a step further. After completing your usual cleaning routine, disinfect your PAP equipment. Use a solution of one part white vinegar to three parts water to soak the tubing, mask, and humidifier chamber for 15 to 20 minutes. This helps kill bacteria and reduce mineral buildup from hard water. Rinse everything thoroughly with clean water to remove any vinegar scent or residue, then air-dry completely.

Check your machine's filter as part of this weekly process. Disposable filters should be replaced according to the manufacturer's instructions, often once a month or sooner if dirty. Reusable filters should be rinsed and dried thoroughly. Keeping filters clean ensures proper airflow and extends the life of your device.

Sterilization Techniques for High-Risk Equipment

For individuals with weakened immune systems, sterilization adds an extra layer of protection. While cleaning and disinfecting are critical, sterilization removes nearly all microbes, including bacteria and viruses. Consider using specialized PAP cleaning machines that employ UV light or activated oxygen to sterilize your equipment. These devices are particularly useful for tubing and other parts that are hard to clean thoroughly by hand.

Alternatively, boiling water can be used to sterilize small, detachable parts like the mask or humidifier chamber, provided they are heat-resistant. Always consult the manufacturer's guidelines before applying heat or sterilization techniques to avoid damaging your equipment.

With consistent care, your PAP equipment will remain a trusted part of your health routine. By dedicating a few minutes each day and following these detailed steps, you can breathe easier—literally and figuratively—knowing your equipment is as clean and safe as it can be.

4

Preventing Cross-Contamination and Maintaining PAP Hygiene

Using PAP equipment is essential for your health, but if not properly maintained, it can unintentionally expose you to harmful germs through cross-contamination. This occurs when bacteria, viruses, or other microbes spread from one surface to another, potentially infecting you or others who come into contact with your equipment. Fortunately, with thoughtful care and preventive measures, you can keep your device safe and hygienic for long-term use.

Understanding Cross-Contamination in PAP Equipment

Cross-contamination can happen in subtle ways. Shared storage areas, handling equipment with unwashed hands, or using improperly cleaned surfaces to dry components can introduce harmful microorganisms to your device. Even small oversights, like not regularly cleaning your humidifier or forgetting to replace a filter, can allow microbes to accumulate and spread.

For individuals with weakened immune systems, the stakes are even higher. Cross-contaminated equipment can lead to infections that are more difficult to fight off. Recognizing these risks is the first step in preventing them.

Best Practices for Preventing Cross-Contamination

To avoid cross-contamination, create a dedicated, clean space for your PAP equipment. Store your mask, tubing, and other components in a covered container or designated drawer to keep them separate from other household items. Wash your hands thoroughly before handling the equipment and after completing the cleaning process.

When cleaning or disinfecting, use tools and materials reserved solely for your PAP equipment—such as a specific brush or cloth—to avoid introducing germs from other sources. Allow your device components to air-dry on a clean surface, like a drying rack or towel designated for this purpose. Avoid using shared towels or sponges, as they can harbor bacteria.

If you have caregivers assisting with your PAP device, ensure they follow proper hygiene protocols. They should wash their hands before and after handling your equipment and use the same cleaning and storage procedures you follow. Consistency in these steps helps minimize risks.

Ensuring Long-Term Maintenance and Hygiene

Keeping your PAP equipment in excellent condition requires more than just routine cleaning—it involves regular inspections and replacements. Over time, components like tubing, masks, and filters can wear down, becoming harder to clean and more susceptible to contamination. Replace these parts according to the manufacturer's recommendations or sooner if they show signs of wear, such as cracks, discoloration, or lingering odors.

Commit to a maintenance schedule that works for you. Daily cleaning, weekly disinfecting, and regular filter changes will keep your equipment functioning properly and prevent cross-contamination. Write down reminders or use a checklist to stay consistent, especially if you're managing other health responsibilities.

By adopting these habits, you're not just maintaining a device— you're safeguarding your health. With clean, well-cared-for equipment, you can focus on the benefits of your therapy and enjoy peace of mind, knowing you've done everything possible to create a safe and healthy environment for yourself and those around you.

5

Recognizing and Responding to Infections from Dirty PAP Equipment

Your PAP equipment is a vital tool for better health, but if it isn't cleaned and maintained regularly, it can become a source of harmful infections. For those with weakened immune systems, the risks are even greater. Recognizing the early signs of an infection and understanding how to manage or prevent them is crucial to staying safe and healthy while using PAP therapy.

Symptoms of Infection from Unclean PAP Equipment

Infections linked to dirty PAP equipment often affect the respiratory system. Symptoms can range from mild to severe and may include persistent coughing, shortness of breath, nasal congestion, or a sore throat. More advanced infections might lead to fever, fatigue, or chest pain. Some individuals may also experience sinus infections or skin irritation around the mask contact points.

Pay attention to any changes in your health, especially if you've been consistent with your PAP therapy. Even minor symptoms can escalate quickly, particularly for individuals with weakened immune defenses. Early detection is the key to addressing infections before they become more serious.

How Dirty PAP Equipment Leads to Infections

The warm, moist environment inside PAP devices, particularly in the tubing and humidifier, provides the perfect breeding ground for bacteria, mold, and viruses. When the equipment isn't cleaned regularly, these microorganisms can build up and circulate through the airflow, entering your respiratory system with every breath.

For example, a humidifier chamber that isn't emptied and dried daily can accumulate stagnant water, where harmful pathogens thrive. Similarly, a dirty filter fails to trap contaminants, allowing them to reach you directly. Over time, the equipment itself can degrade, creating micro-cracks and crevices that are harder to clean and more likely to harbor germs.

Preventing and Managing Infections in Immunocompromised Patients

For those with compromised immune systems, vigilance is critical. Regular cleaning, disinfecting, and sterilizing your PAP equipment significantly reduce the risk of infections. Adhering to a consistent maintenance schedule minimizes the chances of harmful microorganisms taking hold.

If you suspect an infection, contact your healthcare provider immediately. Early intervention can prevent more serious complications. Be prepared to share details about your symptoms, how you've been maintaining your equipment, and whether you've noticed any issues with its condition.

In some cases, healthcare providers may recommend temporary pauses in PAP therapy or adjustments to your routine while addressing the infection. If you're immunocompromised, your care team might also suggest enhanced cleaning protocols or the use of sterilization devices like UV light systems to ensure your equipment remains as safe as possible.

By staying proactive and informed, you can avoid many of the risks associated with PAP equipment. Recognizing the connection between maintenance and health isn't just about following steps—it's about protecting yourself and gaining confidence in your therapy. With clean, well-maintained equipment, you can breathe easy, knowing you've reduced the risks and maximized the benefits of your PAP device.

6

Conclusion

A Lifeline Worth Caring For

Your Positive Airway Pressure (PAP) equipment is more than a machine—it's a partner in your health journey. With its steady stream of air, it helps you breathe easier, sleep better, and live a healthier life. But its effectiveness depends on one thing: proper care. By committing to maintaining your equipment, you're not only safeguarding its performance but also protecting your well-being.

We began by exploring the essential role PAP therapy plays in managing respiratory conditions. This therapy is a lifeline for many, but it also requires respect and responsibility. Without regular cleaning, PAP equipment can harbor harmful pathogens that may lead to serious infections, particularly for those with weakened immune systems.

Next, we delved into the practical steps for cleaning and disinfecting your equipment. A daily routine of washing the mask, tubing, and humidifier chamber, paired with weekly disinfection, is a simple yet powerful way to ensure your device remains safe and effective. For those at higher risk, sterilization techniques provide an extra layer of protection, giving you peace of mind that your equipment is as clean as possible.

Preventing cross-contamination is another vital part of the equation. By creating a clean, dedicated space for your equipment, practicing good hygiene, and using tools reserved solely for maintenance, you can stop the spread of germs before it starts. For caregivers and shared households, these precautions are especially important in protecting everyone's health.

Finally, we discussed the signs of infections caused by dirty PAP equipment and how to respond swiftly and effectively. Recognizing early symptoms, such as coughing, congestion, or skin irritation, allows you to seek help before complications arise. For those with compromised immunity, staying proactive and following enhanced cleaning protocols can make all the difference in preventing serious health risks.

Proper PAP equipment maintenance is not just a routine; it's an act of self-care. It's about taking control of your therapy, minimizing risks, and ensuring that this essential device continues to support you in the best way possible.

By applying what you've learned in this guide, you're investing in your health and well-being. The time and effort you dedicate to cleaning, disinfecting, and caring for your PAP equipment will pay off in better sleep, fewer health complications, and greater confidence in your therapy. Your PAP device is there to help you every night—make sure it's working as it should, free from the risks of neglect.

You deserve to feel safe, supported, and empowered in your journey. With proper care and attention, your PAP equipment can remain a trusted ally, helping you breathe deeply and live fully for years to come.

Thank you for taking the time to read this book. Your commitment to learning about proper PAP equipment maintenance and prioritizing your health is truly inspiring. I hope the information and guidance provided here have given you the tools to care for your equipment and, more importantly, to safeguard your well-being or that of someone you care about.

If you found this book helpful and believe it has added value to your therapy or understanding, I would be truly grateful if you could share your thoughts in a review on Amazon. As your feedback not only helps others discover this resource but also encourages me to continue creating content that supports individuals like you.

Your health journey is important, and it's an honor to have been a small part of it. Thank you for allowing this book to be your guide, and I wish you continued success in your path toward better health and restful nights.